I0412106

# Nature's Miracle Elixir

## The Essential Health Benefits of Coconut Oil

Judith Turnbridge

© 2013 Judith Turnbridge

**All Rights Reserved. No part of this publication may be reproduced in any form or by any means, including scanning, photocopying, or otherwise without prior written permission of the copyright holder.**

Disclaimer and Terms of Use: The Author and Publisher has strived to be as accurate and complete as possible in the creation of this book, notwithstanding the fact that he does not warrant or represent at any time that the contents within are accurate due to the rapidly changing nature of the Internet. While all attempts have been made to verify information provided in this publication, the Author and Publisher assumes no responsibility for errors, omissions, or contrary interpretation of the subject matter herein. Any perceived slights of specific persons, peoples, or organizations are unintentional. In practical advice books, like anything else in life, there are no guarantees of income made. This book is not intended for use as a source of legal, business, accounting or financial advice. All readers are advised to seek services of competent professionals in legal, business, accounting, and finance field.

First Printing, 2013

Printed in the United States of America

# Table of Contents

# Introduction

There's no doubt about it; coconut oil is amazing stuff! It's completely natural, relatively cheap and extremely good for you, as long as it is used sensibly.

For centuries, thousands of people from all over the globe have testified that coconut oil transformed the quality of their lives by providing them with invaluable protection and relief from a bewildering variety of diseases and health issues.

Decades of evidence suggests that the incredibly low levels of heart disease, arthritis, and high-blood pressure encountered among the people of the South Pacific are mainly due to their use of this "magic" oil.

Many celebrities swear by it too. Actress, Angelina Jolie, starts each morning with a spoonful of coconut oil. Gisele Bundchen smothers her body with it, while fellow super-model Miranda Kerr swallows *four tablespoons* of coconut oil every day while using it in her salad dressings, cooking oils, and cups of green tea!

There are many claims that coconut oil is good for the heart, the bowels, the skin, our hair, and even our mental well-being. It is even said to be beneficial to the health of our pets!

Yet, despite all the testimonials and scientific evidence supporting these claims, no other food in modern history has courted so much controversy and confusion.

This book attempts to answer the many questions surrounding this contentious product, by discussing the potential benefits and pitfalls of this humble, yet incredible, food.

Please note however, that although I have thoroughly researched the science surrounding coconut oil and related issues, I am not a medical practitioner nor do I possess bio-chemical qualifications.

(I've included a selected list of references for you to follow at the end of this book that I used during my investigations.)

Therefore, this book is not intended to dispense medical advice. The goal is to simply provide you with the data you need to make informed decisions about this product.

However, before we start, let's find out a little more about what we are actually dealing with here.

# What on Earth Is Coconut Oil Anyway?

Coconut oil is a clear, sticky extract, pressed from the flesh of a coconut. That seems pretty straightforward, but its composition might surprise you.

## What Is Coconut Oil Made Of?

According to the U.S. Department of Agriculture, coconut oil consists of the following:

91% Saturated fatty acids

6%   Mono-unsaturated fatty acids (Oleic Acid)

3%   Poly-unsaturated fatty acids

Yes. You read that correctly; 91% saturated fat! Yikes!

Because of this high percentage, the U.S. Food and Drug Administration suggests limiting the amount you eat in order to minimize the risks associated with excessive saturated fat consumption.

Accordingly, the Coconut Research Center, recommends a maximum daily intake of about 3.5 tablespoons, which, they say, should provide you with all the available health benefits, while avoiding many of the perceived issues. (I believe the FDA is being a little over-cautious about coconut oil. There's much more about this in later chapters so please read on!)

## What Is the Difference Between Coconut Milk, Coconut Oil, and Virgin Coconut Oil?

Contrary to what many people believe, coconut milk is the white, creamy liquid produced from grated coconut meat – not the fluid that fills the cavity of the fruit. This is called the "juice" (no, that wasn't a typo earlier. Technically, coconuts are not a "nut" at all, but a type of fruit known as a "drupe".   Therefore, they share the same food category as peaches, mangoes etc.). Though consisting mainly of water, coconut milk contains a high percentage of oil, which is responsible for its distinctive flavor.

Commercial, mass-produced, coconut oil is pressed from copra.  Copra is the slow-dried flesh of the coconut.

Unfortunately, the drying process contaminates the copra with all kinds of nasty germs and bacteria, so the extract needs to be refined, bleached, and deodorized before it can be consumed – hence the term RBD coconut oil.

RBD coconut oil is refined with Sodium Hydroxide to improve its shelf life (also termed "hydrogenation"), bleached through clay filters to remove any impurities, and passed through high-temperature furnaces for deodorizing. That's a lot processing! Unsurprisingly, the quality of the final product can vary significantly. Moreover, RBD oil is nowhere near as good for you as virgin oil, and may even be bad for you in certain situations due to the hydrogenation procedure (there's more on this in the section on heart disease).

Virgin coconut oil does not use copra, and it is pressed directly from fresh coconut meat. No chemicals, filtering, or heating are used at all in the production process of virgin coconut oil, so it is much purer and healthier oil.

## Capsules or Liquid? What Form of Coconut Oil Should I Use?

Coconut oil can come in handy capsules, but I wouldn't recommend buying them because they are often expensive, and contain ordinary – not virgin – oil. Moreover, they are useless to cook with! For medicinal purposes, simply sip it from a spoon or use it in your food.

## Is There a Way to Keep Coconut Oil from Solidifying?

Coconut oil usually comes in jars or bottles. It tends to solidify at temperatures below 24 degrees Celsius. There is no way to prevent this. It is nothing to worry about, however, as it is not a sign there is anything wrong with the oil or that it has gone rancid.

# The Benefits of Coconut Oil

As mentioned in the introduction, the range of claimed health benefits provided by coconut oil is huge. They include:

– Improved hair and skin care

– Improved dental health and bone strength

– Stress management

– Cholesterol control

– Weight loss

– A strengthened immune system

– Improved digestion and metabolic regulation

– Treatment for kidney problems, heart disease, high blood pressure, diabetes and some types of cancer

That's quite a list!

The oil is so good for you because it contains lauric, capric, and caprylic fatty acids. These all have powerful antimicrobial, antioxidant, antifungal, and antibacterial properties that help combat and prevent decease.

As you can see, coconut oil can be wonderfully good for you. However, since it is mostly composed of saturated fat, which definitely isn't good for you, there could be some concerns.

For decades, health agencies across the world have stated that consuming large quantities of saturated, fatty acids can cause a multitude of potentially fatal conditions, such as coronary heart decease, diabetes, and cancer.

This begs the question:

## How Is Coconut Oil Supposed to be Healthy When It's so Full of Fat?

Sorry, guys but this is where I must get "technical" for a moment. Like they say in the shampoo ads, "Here's the science". Don't be put off by words like "molecule" and fatty acids; this is not as daunting as it looks, I promise!

In a nutshell (excuse the pun), not all fats are equal – at least in terms of the harm they can do to the body.

The saturated fat in coconut oil is composed of a special type of molecule; lauric fatty acid. (Fatty acids are the molecules that make up fat). Not only are they far less harmful than ordinary fatty acids, they actually promote good health.

According to Bruce Fife, N.D. of the Coconut Research Center, the difference is in the length of these fatty acids.

About 98% of all the fats and oils we eat every day are made of great, big long-chain fatty acids (LCFA). Because of their size, they are hard for the body to digest and so initially become stored in the fat-cells. This is the reason butter makes you flabby!

As our bodies struggle to process LCFA's, our "bad" cholesterol levels rise to those beyond which we can cope. Over time, the excess cholesterol builds-up inside us clogging-up and hardening our arteries (atherosclerosis) as well as damaging many of our vital organs. Ultimately, this can lead to heart disease, high-blood pressure, fatty-livers, diabetes, various cancers, and all sorts of horrible, life-threatening illnesses.

However, the lauric acid found in coconut oil has a very different effect on the body, as it is a medium-chain fatty acid (MCFA). (Coconut oil contains a couple more MCFA's, though, at a much lower proportion than lauric acid. Those are capric acid and caprylic acid, which both provide similar health benefiting properties to lauric acid).

MCFA's are much more easily digested than long-chain saturates. They release quick shots of energy when the body processes them, rather than getting stored as fat.

An offshoot of this is, MCFA's won't increase the levels of "bad" cholesterol in your blood stream and may actually help to protect you against both atherosclerosis and heart disease by raising your levels of "good" cholesterol. It's the main reason coconut oil is said to be so good for people. (There's more about this in the chapter on heart disease).

There are very few natural sources of MCFA and the best definitely come from coconut and palm kernel oils. (You won't find them in any cheeseburger...that's for sure!)

## How Else Is Lauric Acid Good for Me?

You want *even more* science knowledge? Wow, you are brave!

When your body processes lauric acid it is converted into monolaurin. Research has demonstrated that monolaurin has powerful antibacterial, antifungal (it's a yeast killer too), and antimicrobial effects in the lab (see references chapter).

Lauric acid attacks and helps kill viruses that have a lipid (fatty) coating, such as herpes, hepatitis, the flu, and mononucleosis.

It also helps ward off harmful bacteria such as listeria monocytogenes and helicobacter pylori, as well as nasty non-cellular parasites such as giardia lamblia.

Although western medicine has been slow to catch on to the health benefits that the lauric acid in coconut oil provides, those in Asia have known about them for centuries. Indeed, it has been one of the corner stones for treatment in Ayurveda; a Hindu traditional Indian medicinal system that is at least 3500 years old!

## Does Coconut Oil Have Any Adverse Side Effects?

In order to get the full benefits, you must take regular doses of up to 3-4 tablespoons of coconut oil a day.

That's a lot of oil!

For the newbie, this can be a little hard on the system. Initial consumption may lead to nausea, vomiting, and even diarrhea. Therefore, the Coconut Research Center suggests that users gradually building up the dosages when starting treatment. Much like many other long-term medications, this will give a person's body the time it needs to adapt to the coconut oil.

## If It's so Good for People, Why Don't More of Us Know About It?

You might not know this, but coconut oil was used fairly regularly in the U.S. for baking, frying, and even making popcorn right up to the beginning of the 1980's.

Then, according to Bruce Fife N.D., the American Soybean Association (ASA) began an orchestrated attack on the reputation of the safety of coconut oil in order to shake public confidence in this product and, as a result, hopefully sell more of their soybean oil. They were soon joined in the 1990's by the Corn Products Company (CPC International), and finally the Centre for Science in the Public Interest (CSPI).

The ASA pushed the line that as saturated fats caused heart disease, coconut oil must also cause heart problems because of its high concentration of it. Ironically, once they got the backing of the CSPI, any scientific detachment went right out the window. Despite a maelstrom of half-baked claims, assumptions, and bogus accusations, the CSPI, inexplicably failed to run any tests!

There were even congressional hearings, but the poorer nations, who exported coconuts, couldn't fight the vast, rich U.S. food industry. All too soon, heart disease rates began to soar. Once the media jumped on the band-wagon, the fate of coconut oil was sealed and its reputation trashed. Almost overnight, partially hydrogenated soybean oil would replace coconut oil and could be found in pretty much everything we eat!

Now this may sound a little like a conspiracy theory and I'd be the first to admit I love a good one of those. After reading Eric Von Däniken's, *Chariots of the Gods?*, back in the 70's, I nearly burst a rib laughing because it was so stupid. Not to mention, what about the Apollo landings? It never ceases to amaze and amuse me that, despite overwhelming evidence, some people still can't believe we actually made it to the Moon. Hopefully, that helps prove that I'm not a natural conspiracy theorist.

Now, what Dr. Fife, and his supporters fail to mention here is that the coconut oil used in the US was the commercial stuff. As this oil was also hydrogenated, it certainly couldn't be live up to the claim of being healthy!

However, despite all the misinformation surrounding this issue, I think Fife might have a point.

First, there is plenty of theoretical evidence suggesting virgin coconut oil is at least benign for the cardiovascular system and may even be good for it. There are literally, hundreds of first-hand testimonials out there supporting this (although space doesn't permit including them all).

There are also several population studies that suggest the virgin oil is good for you. Multiple reports have shown that despite deriving as much as 60 percent of their caloric intake from coconut oil, the residents of the Pacific Islands have almost non-existent rates of cardiovascular disease.

According to various sources, within a decade of India switching from coconut oil to hydrogenated soybean oil the number of deaths caused by heart disease has tripled.

News Medical states that way back in 1994, researchers conservatively estimated that 30,000 Americans died prematurely every year from eating the very similar fats contained in our food. Those figures have almost certainly grown dramatically since then.

So you have to ask yourself, if this hydrogenated stuff is so harmful, then why are there so few alternatives out there? Comparatively, why has so little research been undertaken in the U.S. on the benefits of non-hydrogenated coconut oil, particularly in light of the obesity epidemic now sweeping the nation?

It makes you wonder, doesn't it?

# Hair Care

You probably already know that coconut oil is great for your hair, especially if you've paid any attention to all those commercials for shampoos and conditioners that promote its use.

For centuries, hundreds of millions of the people all over the Indian sub-continent have used coconut oil on their hair each day as they bathed. This shouldn't be too much of a surprise since it is one of the best natural nutrients for your hair.

Coconut oil is a wonderful conditioner, that helps promote healthy hair growth as well as producing a beautiful, glossy shine. It helps strengthen hair, repair damage, and promotes re-growth by providing nourishment and reducing protein loss in hair fibres.

So, without further ado, let's dig a little further into the subject and find out how to use it.

## Coconut Oil Can Make Your Hair Grow Faster, Thicker, Longer, and Less Frizzy!

A research study carried out at Princeton University in 2001 stated that coconut oil provided better hair protection from hygral fatigue – which is technical talk for what makes hair break easily! So how does it work?

If hair is too porous, the continual leakage of water in and out of the fibres causes them to weaken and snap. This results in locks that never seem to grow long and continually looks dull, dry, thin, and wispy (...sounds like a '60's band).

This is where coconut oil comes to the rescue! The tiny molecules in the oil help block these pores and therefore prevent the dreaded hygral fatigue setting in. Your hair will be much thicker and stronger as well as better able to handle the weight-strain from longer strands.

## Coconut Oil Kills Dandruff and Stops Lice (Yuck!)

By regularly massaging your head with coconut oil, you can cure yourself of horrible itchy dandruff, even if your scalp is dry as a bone.

It works so well that it is often used in commercial hair care products, conditioners, and anti-dandruff shampoos.

Even more remarkably, coconut oil can help keep your kids' hair and scalp free from pesky lice and their yucky eggs that thrive on dry hair.

## Should I Use Regular Coconut Oil or Extra-Virgin Coconut Oil on My Hair?

You can use either extra-virgin or unrefined coconut oil for hair and scalp treatments; it doesn't make that much difference. For a little extra nourishment and shine, it's a good idea to add therapeutic-grade essential oils to the mixture. You can find these in most health food stores.

## How to Apply Coconut Oil to Your Hair

**Daily conditioning:** Apply about a 1/8 of a tablespoon of oil to your dampened hair, and then comb it through from the scalp to the ends.

Leave it on and style your hair as you would normally. This comb-in and leave conditioning will add volume and a glossy shine to your hair.

**Deep conditioning:** Shampoo your hair, towel it dry, and then pour a drop of oil about the size of a quarter onto the palm of one hand. Rub both hands together briskly to warm up the oil. Next, run your fingers through your hair, from the roots to tips, to evenly distribute the oil. Keep doing this until all your hair is thoroughly saturated. When finished, cover your head with a shower cap or a clean towel for an hour or so. Lastly, shampoo the oil out of your hair and then style as usual.

Alternately, why not try making your own coconut and sesame oil conditioner! All you need to do is grab a bowl and pour in the following: One tablespoon of coconut oil, two tablespoons of olive oil, and two tablespoons of sesame oil. Then add two teaspoons each of honey and coconut milk. Finally, crack in two eggs. Thoroughly combine the mixture then apply it to your hair from the scalp to the ends. Let it soak for about 20 to 30 minutes, and then shampoo it out.

**Anti-dandruff treatment:** Heat up a tablespoon of coconut oil until it is hot. Then allow it to cool down again until it is comfortable for you to touch. Vigorously, massage it into your scalp, comb out any tangles, then wrap up your head in a towel or shower cap. Leave the oil on overnight, and then in the morning, wash it out with a mild shampoo. (It's a good idea to cover your pillow with a towel just in case the cap or head-towel shifts while you sleep). Repeat this process three times a week until the dandruff is gone.

**Treating a dry, itchy scalp:** Each night before going to bed, part your hair one section at a time and then vigorously apply a small amount of coconut oil to your scalp. Repeat the process until the entire head is done. Next, comb out any tangles you have with a wide-tooth comb and then put on a shower cap. Leave the oil on overnight to work its magic! In the morning, remove the cap and wash it out with a mild shampoo as usual.

Do this daily until your scalp is healthy. It can take up to 5 weeks before the dryness has subsided, but it will certainly be worth the effort.

**Hiding split ends:** Massage approximately 1/4 teaspoon of coconut oil onto the split ends. Then cover them with plastic wrap and leave on overnight. Shampoo the oil out the following morning and then style as usual. Although the coconut oil won't actually repair the split ends, it should make them far less noticeable.

**Making homemade shampoo:** Heat two tablespoons of coconut oil in a saucepan until it is warmed all the way through. Remove the pan from heat and then add a drop of rose and three drops of orange essential oils. Let the mixture cool down for approximately five minutes and then pour it into a glass jar with a screw-top lid. Leave this to harden. To use, simply apply the solidified shampoo to sections of your hair and then comb it through from roots to the tips. When finished, rinse it out thoroughly with hot water.

# Skin Care

As with hair, there are literally hundreds of products out there that use coconut oil for skin care. The use of coconut oil for this purpose long stretches back into history. You've probably used at least one of these on yourself, so you don't need me to tell you how great this stuff can make your skin feel.

Did you know, however, there's also scientific evidence to support this? The Journal of the American Contact Dermatitis Society reports that virgin coconut oil is great for combating the growth of the viruses, fungi, and bacteria that cause skin conditions such as eczema and acne. This means not only can it treat skin problems, but it can also help prevent them too.

Be aware though, that, as coconut oil is antiviral and antifungal, it will actively draw out all the toxins in your skin. An unfortunate side effect of this is that you might notice a few pimples break out for the first couple of weeks you use it. Don't panic because this is actually a good sign! If you stick with the treatment, the spots will soon disappear. In turn, you will be rewarded with beautiful, healthy, glowing skin!

Also be aware that if you experience any severe swelling, redness, or itching after using the oil, your skin may be allergic to it. In that case, it is advisable to stop using it. If you have any concerns, do not hesitate to seek medical advice.

## How to Use Coconut Oil for Skin Care

Before you begin any skin treatment, make sure you only use extra-virgin coconut oil, as commercial coconut oils may contain impurities that can clog your pores. Rub some of it on a small patch of your skin first, to test for allergic reactions. The best places to do this are on delicate areas that are largely out of sight, such as the inside of the forearm or the back of the neck. Obviously, if you do get any sort of reaction, don't use the oil anywhere else on your skin.

## Coconut Oil as a Facial Cleanser

When using coconut oil as a facial cleanser, the first step is to wash your face in warm water only and then pat it dry with a freshly laundered towel.

Next, you need to make the cleanser. For normal skin, mix two tablespoons of castor oil with two tablespoons of coconut oil. If your skin is greasy, use three tablespoons of castor oil to one of coconut. For dry skin, use one tablespoon of castor oil to 3 tablespoons of coconut.

Now, boil up four cups of water in a kettle and pour it into a large bowl. Put this on a table that is the right height for you to comfortably place your face over it and absorb the steam. Once done, gently massage the coconut cleanser into your face and then drape a towel over your head and the bowl. Now lower your face until you are about eight to ten inches above the water.

Sit for 10 minutes to allow the oily vapors to penetrate your facial pores and cleanse the skin. Once the time is over, wipe the oil off your face with a warm, freshly laundered facecloth. Last, you should perform a final rinse-over with lukewarm water.

If you do this once a week, your face will literally be glowing with health. However, be sure not to do this more than three times per week or else you may cause the skin to negatively react.

## Coconut Oil as a Face Mask

If you prefer to make a coconut oil face mask, you begin by mashing up half an avocado in a bowl and then adding half a tablespoon of coconut oil along with a half a tablespoon of honey. A scientific study carried out at Charles Stuart University in Australia demonstrated that honey, like coconut oil, possesses powerful antibacterial and anti-inflammatory properties, making it great for treating skin conditions like acne or eczema.

Now spread this paste over the face and leave it on for 45 minutes. Since the mask is very moist due to the oil, it will not dry up on your skin. This means it can be easily and comfortably removed.

Once the time is up, grab a clean, wet, washcloth or paper towel and wipe off the mask from your face. If there is anything remaining, rinse it off thoroughly with warm water. Make sure the entire mask is cleaned away.

Finally, close the pores by rinsing off your face with lukewarm water.

If done regularly, this coconut mask remedy will leave your skin feeling as smooth and soft as a baby's. As with any facial mask, however, be sure not to apply this more than once a week.

## Coconut Oil as a Moisturizer

After washing your face with a skin cleanser, pat it dry, and then simply take a dab of coconut oil and rub it gently into the skin. This works as a moisturizer and should leave your face feeling soft and smelling great.

## Coconut Oil as an Acne Treatment

First, wash your hands and then your face using a gentle cleanser. Cleaning your hands first helps prevent the spread of viruses and bacteria to the face, which will give the coconut oil less work to do when you apply it. The cleaning will also help to open the pores and allow the oil to be absorbed more easily and thoroughly.

Next, pat your face dry with a clean, dry towel and then lightly rub a thin coat of coconut oil into the skin around evening time. Leave the oil on for 10 to 15 minutes to allow the skin to absorb it and then gently wash the face again with cleanser.

## Coconut Oil for Rashes, Eczema, Psoriasis, or Severe Dryness

For the treatment of these sore blemishes, apply a small dab of oil directly to them, and then cover them with an appropriately sized bandage. Leave the adhesive bandages on overnight, remove in the morning, and then wash your face with a skin cleanser. If you are allergic to the glue on bandages (as I am), you can use dressings applied with strips of non-allergenic surgical tape.

You could simply leave the oily patches exposed to the air, but then you must be very careful to keep them clean by not touching them with your hands. If you do, you may re-infect the skin as well as undo all the good work the oil is doing (and, of course, you'll get your hands smothered in grease). It is important that you keep these areas moistened with the oil, so if you do accidentally wipe any off, re-apply more as soon as you can.

## How Long Does It Take Coconut Oil to Rid Your Skin of Acne and Other Problems?

The short answer is that it depends. Ultimately, the body's immune system defeats these conditions, so the health of the person and the severity of the infections encountered are the key factors here. Consequently, it may take a couple weeks or even up to six months before you notice any real difference, so perseverance with these treatments is a must. As long as you don't expect over-night results, you won't be disappointed. You can improve matters a little, by taking the oil internally as this may strengthen your immune system. (There's more on this later – so keep on reading).

## Coconut Oil as a Natural Sunscreen

Homemade sunscreens with a coconut oil base are not only cheap, but they are also free from the potentially carcinogenic chemicals, such as aluminum zirconium, benzophenones, and salicylates that are found in many commercial alternatives.

Here's how to make the sunscreen. First, add three tablespoons of shea butter to six of coconut oil into a medium bowl and then briskly whip them together using a wire whisk.

Next, add two tablespoons of zinc oxide to the mix and whisk it in. The zinc oxide is a natural "physical" sun-blocking agent that filters out both UVA/UVB rays.

Finally, pour the mixture into a lidded, plastic container and then store it in the refrigerator.

You use this in exactly the same way as any other sunscreens. Simply, rub it into your skin with your fingertips before going outdoors.

## Coconut Oil as a Natural Deodorant

Just like the sunscreen described above, coconut-based homemade deodorants are free of carcinogens and relatively cheap. Plus, it uses one of my favorite, natural, ingredients – baking soda (if this stuff were human, I'd ask for its autograph!).

First, pour a ¼-cup of baking soda along with a similar quantity of corn starch into a medium-sized bowl. Combine the two together with a metal whisk.

Next, add five tablespoons of coconut oil to the mix, along with a few drops of your favorite, scented, essential oil.

Mix all of the ingredients together with the whisk, until a thick paste has formed and then scoop it all into a lidded, plastic container. Store the container in the fridge to keep it fresh.

To use, simply take a quarter-sized drop of the deodorant and rub it into your underarms with your fingertips, whenever you start to smell a little funky under there!


## Coconut Oil as an Exfoliating Facial Scrub


Here is yet another remedy that uses baking soda. All you have to do is mix the soda with an equal quantity of coconut oil and then massage this concoction into your face. Then simply rinse it off with warm water. You can pre-make the scrub and store it in a re-sealable jar.

An alternative "recipe" I recently found on the Internet calls for combining a two to one ratio of brown sugar to coconut oil and then adding a few drops of lavender "to taste". You use it and store it in exactly the same way as mentioned above. I can't personally vouch for its effectiveness, but I'm sure it tastes pretty yummy!

## Coconut Oil to Treat Dark Elbow Patches

Rub a drop of coconut oil onto your elbows once every morning and then again before you go to bed at night until they disappear. This treatment works great!

## Coconut Oil to Treat Nail Fungus

As you might have gathered by now, coconut oil is a naturally powerful anti-fungal agent, so it's great for treating these types of conditions.

For fungal infected nails, merely rub a drop of oil into the nail in the morning and repeat in the evening. Repeat this daily until the infection has subsided (within a week or so, you should notice some sort of improvement, such as less crumbling or a reduction in nail thickness). Remember to wash your hands before and after application to prevent the spread of infection.

## Coconut Oil to Treat Athlete's Foot

Treating athlete's foot is a little more work than nail fungus. In order to treat athlete's foot, you can make your own antifungal cream by mixing one tablespoon of coconut oil with at least five drops of one or a combination of the following oils: tea tree, oregano, garlic, or clove. Rub this cream well into all affected areas of the feet.

Apply the cream at least 20 minutes or so before you go to bed, allowing it to soak in completely before you get into bed. A good idea in order to help you avoid oily bed linens and to keep the cream on is to wrap up your feet with gauze or a clean, white cloth.

You can pre-make this mixture ahead of time and there's no need to refrigerate it.

Soak your feet twice a day in a coconut-based antifungal solution. This is made from a few drops of coconut vinegar (you can get this in many health food stores or online), a clove of crushed garlic, and enough lemon tea to cover the feet. (Make sure the tea is not too scolding hot). The vinegar and lemon in the tea leave a healthy acid layer on your soles that help to combat the infection. The garlic also has powerful anti-fungal properties. (I can feel another book coming on...). Once you've soaked, pat your feet dry with a paper towel and then apply the coconut oil anti-fungal cream mentioned earlier.

Be sure to handle with care and keep both of these solutions out of your eyes! If you do so accidentally get any into your eyes, be sure rinse them well with a solution of one teaspoon of baking soda stirred into a cup of sterile or distilled water. It's a good idea to make this ahead of time in case of an emergency. This solution actually makes great eyewash that you can use anytime and that keeps well in your closet or medicine cabinet.

According to Dr. Fife and the Henry Spink Foundation, fungal conditions may be a symptom of a weakened immune system. This can lead to excessive build-up of yeast, promoting these types of ailments. Therefore, they recommend, taking coconut oil orally to combat any build-ups and to prevent re-occurrences of fungal infections.

## Coconut Oil to Help Erase Stretch Marks

It isn't easy to get rid of stretch marks; I should know. Giving birth, twice, has certainly taken its toll on my body. Fortunately, there are a number of natural remedies out there that can help make them a little less obvious and one of the best is made of coconut oil! (No surprises there!)

This mixture consists of a one to one mix of vitamin E oil to coconut oil. You can purchase vitamin E oil in almost all department stores and health food chains. Simply, rub a little of the mixture into the stretch marks every day and gradually they will fade.

## Coconut Oil Lip Balm

Here's a great recipe to make your own natural lip balm to soften and soothe your chapped lips.

Take a small pot and fill it with the following ingredients: four tablespoons of coconut oil, three tablespoons of sweet almond or apricot kernel oil, two tablespoons of grated beeswax and between five – ten drops of sweet orange oil or any other essential oil of your choice.

Next, over a low heat, gently whisk the pot contents until a runny liquid is formed. Pour this straight into lip-balm tubes or screw-top pots and allow these to cool for at least 20 minutes until the balm has solidified. The amount made here is about ¾ ounce.

Be aware this can be very smelly as it cools down. If this starts to get to you, pour another, thin layer of the mixture over the top, to seal off the fumes.

Remember, to make sure the balm has fully cooled before you use it, though, or else you may burn your lips! (Ok, I did this myself once - Duh!)

# Heart Disease

As mentioned earlier, coconut oil has often had received some bad press and this information is either biased or just, plain misleading. Here's an example:

In the late 1990's, the Center for Science in the Public Interest (CSPI) "red-flagged" America about the health risks posed by the massive doses of saturated fat contained in movie-theater popcorn cooked in coconut oil.

As recently as 2009, they repeated the warning, labeling coconut oil a "heart-stopping fat."

So, if that's true, how can it be "good" for the heart? Confusing isn't it?

It turns out that, regarding health risks and benefits, all saturated fats are not equal the same way that all coconut oils are not equal either! Are you with me? No? Ok, let's try again.

Basically, we're talking about two types of coconut oil here: processed (refined), commercial coconut oil (the baddie), and un-refined, virgin coconut oil (the hero).

According to Cornell University, along with many other sources, hydrogenated fats and oils (commonly called "trans fats"), cause cardiovascular disease. As far as commercial coconut oil goes bad quickly, it needs hydrogenation to increase its shelf life, thus making it bad for your heart.

As movie-theatre popcorn was cooked exclusively in this cheap, "trans-fatted" junk it kicked off the warnings from the CSPI. Unfortunately, these reports failed to make the distinction between virgin coconut oil and the unhealthy commercial rubbish. Therefore, both types of coconut oil "got tarred with the same brush" so to speak.

So, the message here is simple: cheap, commercial oil (or ANY hydrogenated oil for that matter) is bad for your heart, but virgin coconut oil is much better for you.

But, is it actually GOOD for the heart? Let's read on to find out.

## Is Coconut Oil Good for Controlling Cholesterol?

Coconut oil actually INCREASES cholesterol. Huh? Hang on a second! Isn't it this stuff that's going lead to a heart attack or something?

The answer is no! There are two types of cholesterol, one that is good for you and the other that can kill!

Low-Density Lipoprotein (or LDL for short) is the "bad" cholesterol, while High-Density Lipoproteins (HDL) is the "good" stuff.

Even though lauric acid (the "active" ingredient in coconut oil) contains some of the nasty LDL, it actually RAISES your levels of the good, "healthy" HDL.

It's this RATIO of good to bad cholesterol that can influence your chance of getting a heart condition. There are many other factors involved (genetics being one of them), but this is one of the most important.

Moreover, it is suggested that a high ratio of HDL to LDH actually protects the cardiovascular system from disease.

Be aware, however, the research surrounding this phenomenon is patchy at best and more than a little contentious. For instance, at time of this writing, scientists were less than certain that artificially boosting your good cholesterol levels, through taking the oil orally, significantly improved heart health at all.

To further confuse matters, recent research from Texas A&M University suggests that we need a little LDL (the nasty stuff) just to stay alive, calling into question the whole concept of the "cholesterol kills" theory that we've been led to believe was the truth for the past 50 years!

So *is* coconut oil good for cholesterol? It won't lower it, but it can provide a better "balance" of cholesterol in your body. Just be sure to avoid the commercial stuff and use only virgin coconut oil.

As to the question of virgin oil actually being good for the heart, the short answer is "maybe". This is because the ability of this oil to raise 'good' cholesterol in the blood stream is thought to provide protection against cardiovascular disease, even though this has not been conclusively proved *just* yet.

So, what's the "bottom-line"? Coconut oil is certainly no worse for you than any other edible fat, despite the bad press, and in fact, it provides a significantly "safer" alternative to regular cooking oils. Don't go mad with it, and you'll be just fine. Just remember to use only non-hydrogenated, virgin coconut oil and avoid the refined stuff like the plague!

# Weight Loss

As you should know by now, coconut oil contains a special saturated fat called lauric acid that helps "balance" your cholesterol levels and that has loads of other great benefits as well (there's more on these in later chapters). But, did you know that this acid may also help you lose weight?

Now this must seem more than a little counter-intuitive, because even though it's less fattening than many other oils, it's still packed full of calories (about 120 per tablespoon!); which begs another question:

## How Can Coconut Oil Help You Lose Weight if It's so Calorific?

It all comes down to the unique properties of lauric acid.

As mentioned earlier in this book, the medium-chain-fatty-acids that make up this fat are really easy for the body to digest.

Like carbohydrate's, they are burned very quickly by your liver for energy. But unlike most carbs, you won't get an "insulin spike" so they won't contribute to your body's fat-reserves (or the flabby bits as I like to call them – not that you have any, of course!). Also, those nifty little MCFA's boost your metabolism too, so the body is forced to burn your fat reserves for even more energy. The result: a fitter, slimmer you!

Though, known about for centuries in Asia, this phenomenon was first formally reported in the west, way back in the 1940's.

Since coconut oil was very cheap and plentiful back then, farmers tried using it to fatten up their livestock. To their horror, they found it did the opposite! Instead of making the animals fatter, it made them leaner, more active, and even hungrier!

Remember though, that, like all slimming aids, coconut oil is just that; it's an aid to weight loss, not a guarantee. So don't go thinking that by gulping down gallons of the stuff, you can consume cheeseburgers all day and still lose twenty pounds.

The only way anyone can lose weight is for them to burn more calories than they take in.

However, swapping your current cooking fats for coconut oil can certainly make this a lot easier to achieve.

# Crohn's Disease, Inflammatory Bowel Disease, and Other Digestive Problems

Apparently, coconut oil can help to ease the effects of these serious conditions as well as many other digestive problems too! (Is there anything this stuff can't do?)

In fact, physicians at the Naylor Dana Institute for Disease Prevention in Valhalla, New York have so much faith in this natural remedy, they regularly recommend it to patients, for the treatment of such serious and debilitating conditions as Crohn's Disease, irritable bowel syndrome, and ulcerative colitis.

A senior practitioner at the institute, Dr. L.A. Cohen, noted that, as the medium chain fatty acids (MCFA) found in coconut oil are so easily absorbed by the body, it can provide much needed nutrition for suffers of these diseases. As she put it, *"They have found coconut oil to have use in the clinic as a means to provide high energy lipids to patients with disorders of lipid digestion (pancreatitis), lipid absorption (Crohn's disease), and lipid transport (chylomicron deficiency)."*

Moreover, Dr. Cohen and her colleagues are not the only professionals to have faith in the oil. Teresa Graedon, Ph.D., is co-author of *The People's Pharmacy Guide to Herbal and Home Remedies* and an ardent proponent of coconut oil. She states that while researching her book, she encountered so many testimonials on the relief the oil gave to sufferers of Crohn's Disease that she became convinced it was one of the few "home remedies" to have "important medical significance".

One such testimony is from Gerald Brinkley, who has had Crohn's Disease for over three decades. He states, *"When I read that eating coconut macaroons could ease symptoms, I decided to try them myself. Coincidence or not, my symptoms have improved since I began eating two cookies a day."*

Unsurprisingly, Dr. Graedon firmly believes that intensive research needs to be carried out regarding this topic.

You may be wondering by now exactly what Crohn's Disease is, so let me try to enlighten you.

Crohn's Disease is a chronic, inflammatory, intestinal disease which affects approximately 100 to 150 in 100,000 people worldwide. It's a horrible condition, with symptoms that include frequent diarrhea, abdominal cramps, bleeding ulcers, bloody stools, anemia, and severe weight loss. Theses ulcers can occur anywhere along the digestive tract from the mouth all the way down to the rectum.

Ulcerative colitis is a similar chronic disorder, which affects the main colon (the lower part of the intestinal tract). This condition has been linked to increased rates of bowel cancer.

Both conditions are often highly debilitating for sufferers, as they hamper their ability to absorb nutrients into their bodies. This often leads to severe nutritional deficiencies. Sufferers may also find that certain foods aggravate their symptoms, so they have to be constantly wary of what they eat.

Now back to coconut oil!

Besides providing nutrition, the anti-inflammatory and healing properties of coconut oil appear to help soothe inflammation and heal ulceration of the digestive tract.

The fact that studies have shown these benefits is not a recent phenomenon. If fact, researchers have studied and demonstrated these benefits for at least three decades.

The causes of Crohn's Disease and its related conditions are currently unknown. Though a genetic link has been discovered, many doctors believe that a bacterial or viral infection causes these conditions in the same way that the H. pyloris bacterium causes stomach ulcers.

They think this harmful bacteria tunnel their way through the stomach wall, spreading throughout the digestive tract, and resulting in these painful ulcerations.

Many clinical studies have shown that measles and mumps viruses might also be involved.

These studies demonstrate that persistent, low-grade measles infections are common in sufferers of Crohn's Disease and ulcerative colitis.

However, the patients do not show the classic measles symptoms because the infection is "trapped" within their digestive tracts. The evidence for this is pretty convincing, too.

For example, in one study, 36 Crohn's Disease patients, 22 ulcerative colitis patients, and a control group of 89 healthy people were tested for the measles virus. 78% of the Crohn's patients and 59% of the ulcerative colitis patients were found to be infected, while only 3.3% of the control group members carried the virus.

So what does coconut oil have to do with all this?

Lauric acid, the "active ingredient" in coconut oil can kill both H. pylori bacteria as well as the measles virus. If doctors are right, then the symptoms of Crohn's Disease, ulcerative colitis stomach ulcers, and many other related conditions should also be eased when taking the oil.

If you are unlucky enough to have these conditions, you don't have to scoff two coconut macaroons a day as Gerald Brinkley does, to get relief.

Taking the oil neat, or in any recipe rich in it, would work just as well. However, just be sure to eat only virgin coconut oil, so as to avoid the trans-fats and other contaminates in the refined stuff.

## The Very Old, the Very Young, or the Just Plain Sick!

Did you know that for nearly five decades, hospital food and baby formulas have used coconut oil in their recipes? This is because, not only is it full of energy, the special lauric acid within the oil makes it very easy to digest. Therefore, anyone who is too ill to eat properly or who suffers from mal-absorption issues will greatly benefit from it.

This includes very premature babies, cystic-fibrosis suffers, or those with digestive problems.

Lauric acid is so easily digested that it can be almost completely broken down by the salvia and gastric juices alone. Therefore, it only needs a little processing from the pancreas to give off its energy. Coconut oil can subsequently provide quality nutrition for diabetics, the obese, people with gallbladder disease, pancreatitis sufferers, and those with pancreatic insufficiency. It can even provide better nutrition for suffers of certain types of cancer.

As we get older, our pancreases and intestines become less efficient and struggle to keep up with the demands made on them by the rest of the body. This often leads to vitamin deficiencies.

As mentioned earlier, coconut oil requires little processing. As a result, it "frees –up" resources from our digestive systems, allowing them time to "catch-up" and deliver the minerals we need to keep healthy.

When used together with vitamin supplements, foods rich in virgin coconut oil are great for maintaining the fitness levels of the elderly.

# Diabetes and Obesity

Coconut oil can be a great help in preventing and dealing with diabetes, but before we go into the details, let's quickly discover more about this illness.

Diabetes is a disease where the body's pancreas fails to produce enough insulin – the enzyme that helps us to convert the carbohydrates (sugars) from our food into life-giving energy.

This condition is classified into two types:

Insulin Dependent, Type 1 Diabetes is an autoimmune disorder where the body destroys the pancreatic "beta" cells that produce insulin. If untreated, the disease can be fatal and sufferers may need insulin injections throughout their lifetimes to stay alive. About 10 percent of all cases are type 1 diabetic. The cause of this disease has a strong genetic component, with most suffers developing it in early life.

Non-Insulin Dependent, Type 2 Diabetes (formally known as adult-onset diabetes) is a metabolic disorder where, either, the pancreas fails to produce enough insulin or the cells of the body stop responding to it properly (this is termed "insulin resistance"). About 90% of all diabetic cases are type II and most of them develop in adulthood. Though influenced a little by genetics, poor lifestyle is the primary reason an individual becomes a sufferer. Obesity, poor-diet, and lack of exercise are among the most important factors in determining the onset of this condition. Unlike genetics, all of these risk factors are within your control.

## How Coconut Oil Helps Type 2 Diabetes

As mentioned earlier in the "weight loss" chapter, the fat in coconut oil can't be stored in the body, so it is simply burned up and energy is released. This special fat (lauric acid) also helps to speed-up the metabolism. Combined, both factors can contribute to weight reduction.

As obesity is one of the main factors in developing type 2 diabetes, the potential weight reduction brought on by eating coconut oil can help in providing protection from this disease.

Moreover, recent research shows that this isn't the only way the oil benefits type 2 diabetics.

A recent animal study from Australia clearly demonstrates that a diet rich in coconut oil helps to combat the onset of "insulin resistance" (an impaired ability of cells to respond to insulin) in both muscle and fatty tissues.

The study, carried out by Dr. Nigel Turner and Associate Professor Jiming Ye from Sydney's Garvan Institute of Medical Research, shows that the lauric acid in coconut oil increases the "oxidative" (fat burning) capacity of muscle cells, therefore promoting better insulin uptake.

There is a down side, however. Dr. Turner points out, that fat deposits may build up in the liver and therefore advises caution when using it over time. However, this unwanted side effect may be countered by adding other oils to the diet, such as fish oil. The lipids in this are thought to improve the liver's ability to oxidize fat.

So, in a nutshell (I've got to stop using that pun!), for type 2 diabetes sufferers, coconut oil tackles obesity and can help stop the onset of the disease. It also improves the ability for the body to process insulin, which helps with the prevention and management of the condition.

You can substitute coconut oil for the normal oils in your diet, but be sure to combine it with something, like fish oil, to reduce the chance of fat depositing in the liver. As usual, eat only virgin coconut oil to avoid ingesting the harmful trans-fats produced during commercial processing.

## How Coconut Oil Helps Type 1 Diabetes

Coconut oil can provide benefits for type 1 diabetics as well.

The oil's capacity to boost immunity and burn off fat helps to manage the complications that arise from this condition, such as circulatory problems and vulnerability to infection.

As it is crucial for type 1 diabetics to maintain the correct sugar-balance in their blood, coconut oil can provide an easily managed alternative to carbohydrates by providing energy while minimizing insulin demands.

A diet rich in virgin coconut oil and fish oils is recommended. But as always, remember to seek advice from your doctor before embarking on this course. Type 1 diabetes can be very difficult to control and may be life-threatening if it is not managed properly.

# Immunity, Healing, and Infections

You probably knew already that a mother's milk is much better for a child's development than any other type of milk or baby formula.

However, I bet you didn't know that a mother's milk contains more cholesterol than almost any other food! I also bet you didn't know that at least 50 percent of the calories in it come from fat, and most of them are saturated! What is even more remarkable is that the main type of saturated fat found in human milk is our old friend, lauric acid! Yep, that's the same lauric acid found in coconut oil and it plays a vital role in nourishing and protecting babies against infection.

Lauric acid was first found in palm oil by Professor John J. Kabara, from the Department of Chemistry and Pharmacology at Michigan State University, in the 1960's.

Based upon further research by him and many others, Dr. Kabara concluded that because virgin coconut oil contains huge amounts of the stuff, it has anti-viral, anti-bacterial, antifungal, and anti-parasitic properties that "can help control a variety of diseases".

So how does it do this? When processed by the body, the lauric acid in the oil is converted into a substance called "monolaurin". Monolaurin (or 1-Lauroyl-rac-glycerol, to give it its chemical name) has incredible health benefiting properties. Surprisingly, it can be found in many of the things you use daily, such as cosmetics, deodorants, and food additives.

Because of its medicinal properties, many companies now market dietary supplements rich in monolaurin. These products have proved to be incredibly effective across a whole range of diverse applications. Recently, clinics have had considerable success by treating their patients with them. Many top sportsmen take monolaurin to keep their weight down and to improve their athletic prowess. There are even claims that after taking these supplements alone, some HIV suffers experienced huge reductions or improvements in their symptoms.

## What Does Monolaurin Actually Do?

Monolaurin has powerful antibacterial, antiviral, and anti-protozoal properties and it's all due to its chemistry. Cue the science!

In order to easily infect their victims, all harmful bacteria have an unusually weak outer skin made of fatty acids (lipids). Some viruses feature this too. By chance, monolaurin's lipids are the same size as the ones in this skin. Therefore, the bacteria readily absorb it.

Once inside, the monolaurin constantly accumulates. At first, this halts the cells reproductive process. But eventually so much of the stuff builds up inside the bacteria that it literally bursts open like an over-inflated balloon and dies.

Pretty neat trick, huh? It does the same thing to some single celled animals too (protozoa).

Because of this, monolaurin can support the body's immune system in its battle against bugs!

It's quite a selective "magic-bullet" too. The "nice" bacteria constantly live a peaceful co-existence in our bodies and often do valuable jobs, like helping break down stuff in our guts. Monolaurin won't touch these because the skins of the good bacteria are much tougher than the "bad" ones. Therefore, it can't be absorbed by them and bust them apart.

## How Do You Use Monolaurin?

As mentioned earlier, monolaurin can be taken in supplements, but it can also be found in various creams, as well. However, both of these are often expensive. A much cheaper and more versatile alternative is to use virgin coconut oil instead. This is the richest source of lauric acid nature provides. This is a great option since the monolaurin is commercially extracted from coconut oil.

Moreover, although I've never tried, I doubt monolaurin creams are very good to cook with!

## External Applications

When applied to infected skin, coconut oil forms a chemical barrier that seals the area. It also acts as an antiseptic against air-bore "nasties", such as dust particles, fungi spores, bacteria, and viruses.

Coconut oil is also great for treating bruises as it speeds up the healing process by encouraging the repair of damaged tissues.

## Internal Applications

When coconut oil is taken internally, it can be very effective in fighting against a variety of infections. According to the Coconut Research Centre, 3.5 tablespoons of coconut oil per day can help kill the viruses that cause influenza, measles, hepatitis, herpes, SARS, etc. It also kills the bacteria that lead to ulcers, throat infections, urinary tract infections, pneumonia, and gonorrhoea.

Coconut oil is also effective in fighting the fungi and yeast organisms that cause a variety of conditions such as Candida, ringworm, athlete's foot (as covered in the skin care section), thrush, and diaper rash.

# Bone and Dental Health

According to the Coconut Research Center, coconut oil helps improve the body's ability to absorb calcium and magnesium.

This is great news for your teeth and bones.

The enhanced calcium absorption rates help to stop your teeth from decaying and will make them stronger, too! This can help anyone at any age (unless you have dentures), but it is particularly beneficial for your kids.

Together, the increased calcium and magnesium intake is greatly beneficial for middle-aged women who suffer from brittle-bones disease (osteoporosis).

# Stress Relief

Has your son just backed your car into a fire hydrant? Has the dog just chewed your brand new pair of Jimmy Choo's into strips of soggy leather? Has your teenage daughter just decided to run off with a vacuum cleaner salesman from Milwaukee?

Now you could tear your hair out or grab a blunt object and club someone or something to death with it. But why not try something a little less dramatic instead? Grab a bottle of coconut oil and have a bath!

Coconut oil is very soothing and so it is great for freeing you from all the pressures of a stressful day.

Gently massage the oil in a circular motion into your scalp. This is good for promoting circulation and relieving those troublesome stress headaches.

Before going to bed, try pouring a little coconut oil into your nightly bath. This is a fantastic way to un-wind and it will leave your skin silky smooth to boot!

# Moderate Stage Alzheimer's

It has been estimated that over 5 million Americans have been diagnosed with Alzheimer's. The number of those inflicted with this terrible degenerative brain disease is expected to rise massively as our life-spans increase and the population rises.

Up until now, there has been no cure and little effective treatment for the condition. Sufferers were sentenced to a slow, undignified decline, and eventual death.

Recent events suggest, however, there might be some hope for us after all.

When her husband, Steve, developed Alzheimer's, Dr. Mary Newport (a physician from Tampa, Florida) decided not to accept defeat. She researched the subject as much as she could and concluded that the disease was in fact a type of "diabetes of the brain". Realizing the potential benefits, Dr. Newport decided to feed coconut oil to her husband as a treatment. To her amazement, Steve's mental decline was not only halted – it actually went into a sharp reverse. He was able to handle tasks and do other things that would have been unimaginable just a few months before.

Now one swallow does not make a summer, but when she published a book on the subject, Alzheimer's Disease: *What If There Was A Cure?*, Dr. Newport was overwhelmed with "thank you" letters from readers who had tried her method and found similar improvements in their loved-ones.

In my opinion, this is a very promising and interesting development. However, since this has happened so recently, we must be cautiously optimistic. So far, no scientific studies have been conducted on this topic.

Moreover, the cause of Alzheimer's is unknown and Dr. Newport's assertions are – to say the least – controversial.

My take on it is this: the prognosis for this disease is so appalling, that there is little to lose by treating this condition with coconut oil – just try not to invest too much hope in its effects at this time.

# Pet Care

Did you know our furry, four legged friends can also benefit from coconut oil? (I meant your dog – not your horse – tusk!)

In a nutshell (Sorry, I just had to use that again), all the benefits you get from taking this stuff, your dog can get too!

Pups get many growth-benefits from feeding them the oil and most dogs love the taste, making it one of the easiest supplements to feed them.

For best results add it to their food and use it on their bodies. As it is very slow absorbing, you can give your doggy a massage to help it soak in, which of course they'll love!

There are other benefits for dogs too:

– It kills that yucky doggy-pong by adding a drop of coconut oil into their water at bath time.

– Use it as doggy toothpaste! (You've got to be quick with it, though, as they will lick it off the brush.)

– Uses it as a canine skin-cream. It's great for allergies, dermatitis, flaky skin, itchy skin, and it can help heal sores.

– Use it as a coat conditioner. It produces a super shiny coat without the expense.

– Soften and soothe their dry, cracked paws with the oil.

– Banish that belly! Coconut oil helps them lose weight just like it can for humans.

– Use it to detox their bodies. This is especially important if your dog has been eating from your garbage cans!

– Coconut oil can also help with arthritis, sore joints, thyroid problems, and digestive issues. It also prevents and kills yeast infections, ear infections, and viral infections.

As with people, feed only virgin coconut oil to your dog.

Start at half teaspoon a day for each 20 pounds of body weight. However, do not give it all in one dose at first. Instead, give it in small doses throughout the day.

Gradually work up to a full teaspoon, once or twice a day for a 20 pound animal.

If your dog doesn't seem to be feeling well or has loose or greasy looking stools, cut back on the oil for a few days.

Remember that coconut oil detoxes the body, so you'll to need feed it in very small doses so your pet doesn't feel the effects all at once.

# Cooking

This book isn't a cookbook (there are already plenty out there), but this section briefly answers some common questions about cooking with coconut oil.

## Does Coconut Oil Give Food a Slight Coconut Flavor?

The short answer is "yes", although it tastes great on anything sweet or on food that benefits from a subtle coconut flavoring, such as raisin bread, French toast, cookies, brownies, etc.

If you want to fry something savory, then you can completely kill the aftertaste by simply adding a little lemon, lime-juice, or white vinegar to the oil as you cook. It works like magic!

## How Do I Remove the Smell from Coconut Cooking Oil?

See above! Also, make sure you're not over-heating the oil as this can make it smell pretty funky! This is especially true if you're using a steel or copper bottomed pan as these have a tendency to hold in the heat.

## How Much Coconut Oil Is Okay to Eat?

There is no recommended dose of coconut oil, but Pacific Islanders' consume at least one tablespoon daily with no ill effects. The Coconut Research Center suggests taking up to 3.5 tablespoons daily as an appropriate dose. Certified Nutritional Counselor Brian Shilhavy suggests you can safely consume up to four tablespoons daily, but only if you're not counting calories and you have normal cholesterol levels.

## How Do You Use Coconut Oil in Place of Vegetable Oil in Cakes?

Simply use the same amount of coconut oil as you would use of vegetable oil. However, make sure that once it's melted all the other ingredients (eggs, liquids, etc.) are at room temperature or at least warm enough so that the coconut oil doesn't cool down and re-solidify.

You can also use coconut oil in place of shortening.

For every cup of shortening contained in a recipe, you can substitute it for a half-cup of butter and 3/8th of a cup of coconut oil.

## Conclusion

When writing this book I was stunned by how controversial this topic could be. Even more so, I was surprised at just how confusing and often contradictory basic nutritional information is for even the most common foods.

Personally, I get the impression that science cannot really say what is or what isn't good for you – the human body is just too complex and there are too many commercial interests to ensure genuinely unbiased research is performed in these matters.

However, we've now come to the end of our journey, and I sincerely hope you are at least a little clearer as to what coconut oil is and what it can do for you.

Despite the bad press, it is certainly no worse for you than any other oils and there is a mountain of genuine evidence that suggests that, if it is used sensibly, coconut oil is profoundly good for you, your family, and even your dog!

Oh, and by the way, it tastes great when used in cooking too!

I want to finally leave with a quote from my mom:

> "A little of what you fancy does you good".

In the case of coconut-oil that couldn't be more apt!

# References

– Preuss, HG; Echard, B; Enig, M; Brook, I; Elliott, TB (2005). "Minimum inhibitory concentrations of herbal essential oils and monolaurin for gram-positive and gram-negative bacteria". Molecular and cellular biochemistry 272 (1-2): 29–34. PMID 16010969.

– Carpo, BG; Verallo-Rowell, VM; Kabara, J (2007). "Novel antibacterial activity of monolaurin compared with conventional antibiotics against organisms from skin infections: an in vitro    study". Journal of drugs in dermatology: JDD 6 (10): 991–8. PMID 17966176.

– Isaacs, CE (2001). "The antimicrobial function of milk lipids". Advances in nutritional research (10): 271–85. PMID 11795045.

– Lieberman, Shari; Enig, Mary G.; Preuss, Harry G. (2006). "A Review of Monolaurin and Lauric Acid: Natural Virucidal and Bactericidal Agents". Alternative and Complementary Therapies    12 (6): 310. doi:10.1089/act.2006.12.310.

– Projan, S. J.; Brown-Skrobot, S.; Schlievert, P. M.; Vandenesch, F.; Novick, R. P. (1994). "Glycerol monolaurate inhibits the production of beta-lactamase, toxic shock toxin-1, and other staphylococcal exoproteins by interfering with signal transduction". Journal of bacteriology 176 (14): 4204–4209. PMC 205630. PMID 8021206.

– "Microbicide protects monkeys from HIV-like virus". Nature. 4 March 2009. doi:10.1038/news.2009.135.

– http://www.news-medical.net/health/What-is-Trans-Fat.aspx

– Ruetsch SB, Kamath YK, Rele AS, Mohile RB. TRI/Princeton, Princeton, NJ 08540, USA. "Secondary ion mass spectrometric investigation of penetration of coconut and mineral oils into human hair fibers: relevance to hair damage". PMID 11413497

–
http://hcd2.bupa.co.uk/fact_sheets/html/fungal_skin_infections.html

– http://www.raysahelian.com/athletesfoot.html

–Trowbridge, John Parks, M.D., The Yeast Syndrome, New York, New York, Bantam Books, 1986, p. 312-313.

– Novel antibacterial and emollient effects of coconut and virgin olive oils in adult atopic dermatitis. Verallo-Rowell VM, Dillague KM, Syah-Tjundawan BS. Skin and Cancer Foundation, Pasig, Philippines.

– Science Daily  (May 8, 2011) — 'Bad' Cholesterol Not as Bad as People Think, Study Shows

– Steve Riechman, Department of Health and Kinesiology, Texas A&M University
http://www.sciencedaily.com/releases/2011/05/110505142730.htm and the Journal of Gerontology.

– Kaunitz H, Dayrit CS. Coconut oil consumption and coronary heart disease. Philippine Journal of Internal Medicine, 1992;30:165-171

– Prior IA, Davidson F, Salmond CE, Czochanska Z. Cholesterol, coconuts, and diet on Polynesian atolls: a natural experiment: The Pukapuka and Tokelau Island studies, American Journal of Clinical Nutrition, 1981;34:1552-1561.

– Raymond Peat Newsletter, Coconut Oil, reprinted at www.heall.com. http://www.heall.com/body/healthupdates/food/coconutoil.html  An Interview With Dr. Raymond Peat, A Renowned Nutritional Counselor Offers His Thoughts About Thyroid Disease

– Baba, N 1982.Enhanced thermogenesis and diminished deposition of fat in response to overfeeding with diet containing medium-chain triglycerides, Am. J. Clin. Nutr., 35:379

– Dr. Mary G. Enig, Ph.D., F.A.C.N. Source: Coconut: In Support of Good Health in the 21st Century

– Isaacs CE, Litov RE, Marie P, Thormar H. Addition of lipases to infant formulas produces antiviral and antibacterial activity, Journal of Nutritional Biochemistry, 1992;3:304-308.

– Isaacs CE, Schneidman K. Enveloped Viruses in Human and Bovine Milk are Inactivated by Added Fatty Acids(FAs) and Monoglycerides(MGs), FASEB Journal, 1991;5: Abstract 5325, p.A1288.

– Mitsuto Matsumoto, Takeru Kobayashi, Akio Takenakaand Hisao Itabashi. Defaunation Effects of Medium Chain Fatty Acids and Their Derivatives on Goat Rumen Protozoa, The Journal of General Applied Microbiology, Vol. 37, No. 5 (1991) pp.439-445.

– St-Onge MP, Jones PJ. Greater rise in fat oxidation with medium-chain triglyceride consumption relative to long-chain triglyceride is associated with lower initial body weight and greater loss of subcutaneous adipose tissue, International Journal of Obesity & Related Metabolic Disorders, 2003 Dec;27(12):1565-71. http://www.ncbi.nlm.nih.gov/pubmed/12975635

– Geliebter, A 1980. Overfeeding with a diet of medium-chain triglycerides impedes accumulation of body fat, Clinical Nutrition, 28:595

– Fushiki, T and Matsumoto, K Swimming endurance capacity of mice is increased by consumption of medium-chain triglycerides, Journal of Nutrition, 1995;125:531.

# About the Author

Judith Turnbridge is a married artist with an interest in interior design. She enjoys painting, calligraphy, and caring for her garden. Her two children have now grown up and flown the nest, and the two hungry mouths she now feeds belong to her two fluffy cats.

Other books by Judith Turnbridge:

**Super Simple Home Cleaning:** The Best House Cleaning Tips for Green Cleaning the Home

**The Super Simple 30-Day Home Cleaning Plan:** Making Time to Beat the Grime

**How to Organize Your Life to Maximize Your Day:** Effective Time Management Tips and Ideas to Simplify Your Life

**How to Declutter Your Home for Simple Living:** Decluttering Tips and Closet Organization Ideas for Creating Your Own Personal Oasis

**Out of Sight, Out of Mind:** Easy Home Organization Tips and Storage Solutions for Clutter-Free Living

**How to Survive a Disaster:** Emergency Preparedness for You and Your Family

www.ingramcontent.com/pod-product-compliance
Lightning Source LLC
Chambersburg PA
CBHW070623290526
45790CB00002B/963